Borderline Personality Disorder

Ashu Kumawat

Table of contents:

What is Borderline Personality Disorder?

Borderline personality disorder (BPD) is a complex and often misunderstood mental health condition. It is a type of personality disorder that affects a person's thoughts, feelings, behaviours, and relationships with others. People with BPD experience intense and unstable emotions, have difficulty regulating their emotions, and struggle to form stable relationships.

The exact cause of BPD is unknown, but it is believed to be a combination of genetic and environmental factors. People with BPD often have a history of trauma or abuse, such as emotional, physical, or sexual abuse. They may also have a family history of mental health conditions, including BPD.

One of the most defining characteristics of BPD is the intense emotional experiences that people with this condition have. They may experience extreme feelings of emptiness, loneliness, and despair, and may struggle to cope with these emotions in healthy ways. They may also experience intense anger, anxiety, and fear, and may have difficulty calming down once they are upset.

Another common feature of BPD is difficulty with relationships. People with BPD may have a fear of abandonment, and may go to great lengths to avoid being alone. However, they may also push others away or become highly critical of their loved ones, leading to a pattern of unstable and tumultuous relationships. They may also struggle with their own sense of identity, feeling unsure of who they are or what they want out of life.

BPD is a highly stigmatized and misunderstood condition, and people with BPD often face significant challenges in accessing effective treatment and support. However, with the right treatment, people with BPD can learn to manage their symptoms and lead fulfilling lives.

The diagnosis of BPD is typically made by a mental health professional, such as a psychiatrist or psychologist. They will typically use a combination of interviews, questionnaires, and other assessments to evaluate a person's symptoms and determine whether they meet the criteria for BPD.

Some of the criteria used to diagnose BPD include:

Frantic efforts to avoid real or imagined abandonment.

A pattern of unstable and intense interpersonal relationships.

Identity disturbance, such as a sense of self that is unstable or shifting.

Impulsivity in at least two areas that are potentially harmful (such as substance use, reckless driving, or binge eating).

Recurrent suicidal behavior, gestures, or threats, or self-mutilating behavior.

Affective instability, such as frequent and intense mood swings or chronic feelings of emptiness.

Chronic feelings of emptiness or boredom.

Inappropriate, intense anger or difficulty controlling anger.

Paranoia or dissociative symptoms, such as feeling disconnected from oneself or the world.

It is important to note that not all people with BPD will experience all of these symptoms, and that symptoms can vary in severity from person to person.

Treatment for BPD typically involves a combination of psychotherapy and medication. One of the most effective forms of therapy for BPD is dialectical behavior therapy (DBT), which is a type of cognitive-Behavioural therapy that focuses on teaching skills for emotion regulation, interpersonal effectiveness, distress tolerance, and mindfulness. DBT has been shown to be highly effective for reducing symptoms of BPD and improving overall functioning.

Other types of therapy that may be helpful for BPD include cognitive-Behavioural therapy (CBT), psychodynamic therapy, and group therapy. Medications may also be used to help manage symptoms of BPD, such as antidepressants, mood stabilizers, and antipsychotics.

Understanding the Diagnostic Criteria for BPD

Understanding the diagnostic criteria for borderline personality disorder (BPD) can be a helpful tool in understanding the symptoms and experiences associated with this condition. The Diagnostic and Statistical Manual of Mental Disorders (DSM-5) provides a set of criteria for the diagnosis of BPD.

To meet the diagnostic criteria for BPD, a person must experience a persistent pattern of instability in interpersonal relationships, self-image, and affect, as well as marked impulsivity across a variety of areas. The following are the specific diagnostic criteria for BPD according to the DSM-5:

Frantic efforts to avoid real or imagined abandonment: People with BPD may feel intense fear of abandonment or rejection, and may engage in extreme behaviours to avoid being left alone, such as clinging to others or becoming highly dependent on them.

A pattern of unstable and intense interpersonal relationships: People with BPD may have difficulty forming and maintaining stable relationships, often due to their intense and unstable emotions. They may have a history of stormy relationships and frequent breakups.

Identity disturbance: People with BPD may have a persistent sense of emptiness or lack of identity, and may struggle to understand who they are or what they want out of life. They may also experience rapid shifts in self-image and goals.

Impulsivity in at least two areas that are potentially harmful: People with BPD may engage in impulsive behaviours that can be harmful to themselves or others, such as substance use, reckless driving, binge eating, or risky sexual behavior.

Recurrent suicidal behavior, gestures, or threats, or self-mutilating behavior: People with BPD may experience intense feelings of hopelessness and despair, and may engage in suicidal or self-harming behaviours as a way of coping with these emotions.

Affective instability: People with BPD may experience intense and rapidly shifting emotions, such as anger, anxiety, sadness, and elation. They may also have difficulty regulating their emotions and may be prone to intense and prolonged emotional reactions.

Chronic feelings of emptiness: People with BPD may experience a persistent sense of emptiness or boredom, and may struggle to find meaning or purpose in their lives.

Inappropriate, intense anger or difficulty controlling anger: People with BPD may experience intense and unpredictable outbursts of anger, and may have difficulty controlling their anger in certain situations.

Paranoia or dissociative symptoms: People with BPD may experience dissociative symptoms, such as feeling disconnected from oneself or the world, or may experience paranoia or other forms of cognitive distortion.

It is important to note that not all people with BPD will experience all of these symptoms, and that the severity of symptoms can vary widely from person to person. Additionally, some symptoms of BPD, such as impulsivity and affective instability, can also be present in other mental health conditions.

The diagnosis of BPD is typically made by a mental health professional, such as a psychiatrist or psychologist, based on a comprehensive evaluation of the person's symptoms and history. The diagnostic process may include interviews, questionnaires, and other assessments to determine whether the person meets the criteria for BPD.

It is important to remember that a diagnosis of BPD is not a label or a judgment, but rather a tool to help people understand and manage their symptoms. With the right treatment and support, people with BPD can learn to manage their symptoms and lead fulfilling lives.

If you believe that you may be experiencing symptoms of BPD, it is important to seek help from a mental health professional. A therapist or psychiatrist can help you better understand your symptoms, develop coping strategies, and find effective treatment options that work for you. Additionally, there are a number of self-help strategies that you can use to manage your symptoms.

Myths and Misconceptions About BPD

Borderline Personality Disorder (BPD) is a complex and often misunderstood mental health condition. Unfortunately, many myths and misconceptions exist about BPD, which can make it difficult for people with this condition to seek treatment and get the support they need. In this chapter, we will explore some of the most common myths and misconceptions about BPD, and provide accurate information to help dispel these misunderstandings.

Myth: People with BPD are manipulative and attention-seeking.

One of the most pervasive myths about BPD is that people with this condition are manipulative and attention-seeking. This belief is often based on the stereotype of the "dramatic" and "needy" person with BPD, who is constantly seeking attention and causing conflict.

In reality, people with BPD are not intentionally manipulative or attention-seeking. Their behaviours and emotions are often driven by intense fear of abandonment, self-doubt, and a sense of emptiness or lack of identity. They may engage in behaviours such as self-harm or substance use as a way of coping with these intense emotions, but this is not a deliberate attempt to manipulate or control others.

Myth: BPD is not a real or serious mental health condition.

Another common myth about BPD is that it is not a real or serious mental health condition. Some people believe that BPD is simply a "personality flaw" or a result of a person's upbringing or life experiences.

In reality, BPD is a legitimate and serious mental health condition that can have a significant impact on a person's life. People with BPD often experience intense emotional pain, including feelings of emptiness, worthlessness, and hopelessness. They may also struggle with relationships, self-image, and impulse control, and may be at an increased risk for suicide.

Myth: BPD only affects women.

While it is true that BPD is more commonly diagnosed in women than men, this does not mean that only women can have this condition. In fact, research suggests that BPD is just as common in men as it is in women, but may be underdiagnosed in men due to social and cultural expectations around masculinity and emotional expression.

Myth: People with BPD cannot get better or recover.

Another myth about BPD is that people with this condition cannot get better or recover. Some people believe that BPD is a chronic and untreatable condition, and that people with BPD will always struggle with their symptoms and behaviours.

In reality, many people with BPD can and do recover with the right treatment and support. Treatments such as Dialectical Behavior Therapy (DBT) and Cognitive Behavioural Therapy (CBT) have been shown to be effective in helping people with BPD manage their symptoms and improve their quality of life. Additionally, medication may be used to address specific symptoms, such as anxiety or depression.

Myth: BPD is caused by bad parenting or a traumatic childhood.

Finally, a common myth about BPD is that it is caused by bad parenting or a traumatic childhood. Some people believe that people with BPD are simply "acting out" as a result of their upbringing or life experiences.

In reality, the causes of BPD are complex and multifaceted. While a traumatic childhood or difficult life experiences may contribute to the development of BPD, there is no one single cause of this condition. Genetics, brain chemistry, and environmental factors may all play a role in the development of BPD.

In conclusion, there are many myths and misconceptions about BPD that can make it difficult for people with this condition to seek help and get the support they need. By understanding the true nature of BPD, we can work to dispel these misunderstandings and promote greater understanding and empathy for people with this condition.

Causes and Risk Factors for BPD

Borderline Personality Disorder (BPD) is a complex mental health condition that is believed to be caused by a combination of genetic, environmental, and biological factors. In this chapter, we will explore some of the causes and risk factors that may contribute to the development of BPD.

Genetics

Research suggests that there may be a genetic component to the development of BPD. Studies have shown that people with BPD are more likely to have family members who also have the condition, and that identical twins are more likely to both have BPD than non-identical twins.

However, genetics alone are not enough to cause BPD. It is believed that other factors, such as environmental and psychological factors, may interact with genetic predispositions to increase the risk of developing BPD.

Environmental Factors

Environmental factors, such as early childhood experiences, may also contribute to the development of BPD. Traumatic experiences, such as physical or emotional abuse, neglect, or abandonment, can disrupt a child's sense of safety and security, leading to the development of maladaptive coping mechanisms and difficulty regulating emotions.

Children who grow up in unstable or unpredictable environments may also be at increased risk for BPD. For example, children who experience frequent moves, changes in caregivers, or parental substance use may struggle with developing a stable sense of identity and attachment, which can contribute to the development of BPD.

Biological Factors

Finally, there may be biological factors that contribute to the development of BPD. Research suggests that people with BPD may have differences in brain structure and function, including abnormalities in the areas of the brain responsible for regulating emotions and impulsivity.

Additionally, abnormalities in the levels of certain neurotransmitters, such as serotonin and dopamine, have been observed in people with BPD. These neurotransmitters play a role in regulating mood, emotion, and behavior, and imbalances may contribute to the development of BPD symptoms.

Risk Factors

In addition to the causes of BPD, there are also several risk factors that may increase a person's likelihood of developing the condition. These risk factors include:

Trauma or abuse: People who have experienced physical or emotional abuse, neglect, or trauma are at increased risk for developing BPD.

Family history: People who have a family member with BPD are at increased risk for developing the condition themselves.

Childhood environment: People who grew up in unstable or unpredictable environments, such as those with frequent moves or changes in caregivers, may be at increased risk for BPD.

Mental health conditions: People who have other mental health conditions, such as depression, anxiety, or substance use disorders, may be at increased risk for BPD.

Personality traits: People who have certain personality traits, such as impulsivity, emotional instability, or difficulty regulating emotions, may be at increased risk for BPD.

It is important to note that having one or more of these risk factors does not necessarily mean that a person will develop BPD. However, understanding these risk factors can help identify individuals who may be at increased risk and may benefit from early intervention and support.

In conclusion, the causes and risk factors for BPD are complex and multifaceted. While genetics, environmental factors, and biological factors may all play a role in the development of BPD, it is likely that the condition is caused by a combination of these factors. By understanding the causes and risk factors for BPD, we can work to better identify individuals who may be at risk and provide early intervention and support to promote better outcomes.

Differentiating BPD from Other Mental Health Disorders

Borderline Personality Disorder (BPD) shares many symptoms and characteristics with other mental health disorders, which can make it difficult to differentiate and diagnose. In this chapter, we will explore some of the key differences between BPD and other mental health disorders.

Depression

Depression is a common mental health disorder that shares some similarities with BPD. Both conditions can involve feelings of sadness, hopelessness, and worthlessness. However, there are some key differences between depression and BPD.

One of the main differences is in the duration and intensity of symptoms. People with BPD may experience rapid and intense shifts in mood, whereas depression symptoms tend to be more consistent over time. Additionally, people with BPD may engage in impulsive or reckless behavior, which is not typically seen in depression.

Anxiety

Anxiety is another mental health disorder that can share some symptoms with BPD. Both conditions can involve feelings of fear, worry, and panic. However, there are some key differences between anxiety and BPD.

One of the main differences is in the focus of the symptoms. In anxiety, the symptoms are primarily focused on fears and worries related to specific situations or objects. In BPD, the symptoms are more related to fears of abandonment and a lack of stable identity.

Additionally, people with BPD may engage in impulsive or reckless behavior as a way of coping with their symptoms, whereas people with anxiety tend to avoid situations that trigger their anxiety.

Bipolar Disorder

Bipolar Disorder is a mood disorder that shares some similarities with BPD. Both conditions can involve intense mood swings and impulsive behavior. However, there are some key differences between bipolar disorder and BPD.

One of the main differences is in the duration of the mood episodes. In bipolar disorder, mood episodes typically last for weeks or months, whereas in BPD, mood shifts can occur rapidly and unpredictably.

Additionally, people with BPD may experience chronic feelings of emptiness and a lack of stable identity, which is not typically seen in bipolar disorder.

Schizophrenia

Schizophrenia is a serious mental health disorder that shares some symptoms with BPD. Both conditions can involve paranoia, hallucinations, and disordered thinking. However, there are some key differences between schizophrenia and BPD.

One of the main differences is in the severity and duration of symptoms. Schizophrenia symptoms tend to be more severe and persistent over time, whereas BPD symptoms may be more episodic and fluctuating.

Additionally, people with BPD may experience intense feelings of emptiness and a lack of stable identity, which is not typically seen in schizophrenia.

Eating Disorders

Eating disorders, such as anorexia and bulimia, can share some symptoms with BPD. Both conditions can involve a distorted body image, self-harm behaviours, and impulsivity. However, there are some key differences between eating disorders and BPD.

One of the main differences is in the focus of the symptoms. Eating disorders are primarily focused on food and weight, whereas BPD symptoms are related to fears of abandonment and a lack of stable identity.

Additionally, people with BPD may engage in impulsive or reckless behavior as a way of coping with their symptoms, whereas people with eating disorders tend to engage in restrictive or purging behaviours related to their weight and body image.

In conclusion, BPD shares some symptoms and characteristics with other mental health disorders, which can make it difficult to differentiate and diagnose. However, by understanding the key differences between BPD and other disorders, clinicians can make more accurate diagnoses and provide appropriate treatment and support to those who need it.

Diagnosis and Assessment of BPD

The diagnosis and assessment of Borderline Personality Disorder (BPD) can be a complex process, as it involves a thorough evaluation of a person's history, symptoms, and behaviours. In this chapter, we will explore the key components of the diagnosis and assessment process for BPD.

Diagnostic Criteria

The American Psychiatric Association's Diagnostic and Statistical Manual of Mental Disorders (DSM-5) is the primary reference used to diagnose BPD. According to the DSM-5, a person must meet at least five of the following criteria to be diagnosed with BPD:

Frantic efforts to avoid real or imagined abandonment.

A pattern of unstable and intense interpersonal relationships, characterized by alternating between extremes of idealization and devaluation.

Identity disturbance: markedly and persistently unstable self-image or sense of self.

Impulsivity in at least two areas that are potentially self-damaging (e.g., spending, sex, substance abuse, reckless driving, binge eating).

Recurrent suicidal behavior, gestures, or threats, or self-mutilating behavior.

Affective instability due to a marked reactivity of mood (e.g., intense episodic dysphoria, irritability, or anxiety, usually lasting a few hours and only rarely more than a few days).

Chronic feelings of emptiness.

Inappropriate, intense anger or difficulty controlling anger (e.g., frequent displays of temper, constant anger, recurrent physical fights).

Transient, stress-related paranoid ideation or severe dissociative symptoms.

Assessment

The assessment of BPD involves a comprehensive evaluation of a person's history, symptoms, and behaviours. The assessment process may include:

Clinical interview: A clinician will conduct a thorough interview with the person to gather information about their symptoms, behaviours, and history.

Diagnostic testing: Various diagnostic tests may be administered to help identify BPD and rule out other mental health disorders.

Behavioural observations: A clinician may observe the person's behaviors and interactions with others to assess their social and emotional functioning.

Self-report questionnaires: The person may be asked to complete questionnaires or surveys to assess their symptoms and emotional state.

Family history: A clinician may gather information about the person's family history of mental health disorders, substance abuse, or other relevant factors.

Treatment Planning

Once a diagnosis of BPD has been established, the next step is to develop a comprehensive treatment plan. Treatment for BPD typically involves a combination of psychotherapy, medication, and support from family and friends.

Psychotherapy: The most effective treatment for BPD is psychotherapy, which involves working with a mental health professional to develop coping skills, manage emotions, and improve relationships. Different types of psychotherapy that may be helpful for BPD include Dialectical Behavior Therapy (DBT), Cognitive Behavioural Therapy (CBT), and Psychodynamic Therapy.

Medication: While there is no specific medication for BPD, medications such as antidepressants, mood stabilizers, and antipsychotics may be helpful in managing symptoms such as depression, anxiety, and mood swings.

Support from family and friends: BPD can be a challenging condition for both the person with the disorder and their loved ones. Support from family and friends can be instrumental in helping the person manage their symptoms and improve their overall functioning.

In conclusion, the diagnosis and assessment of BPD involves a comprehensive evaluation of a person's history, symptoms, and behaviours. Once a diagnosis has been established, a comprehensive treatment plan can be developed that includes psychotherapy, medication, and support from family and friends. By addressing the underlying issues related to BPD, people can learn to manage their symptoms, improve their functioning, and lead more fulfilling lives.

Comorbid Disorders Associated with BPD

Borderline Personality Disorder (BPD) is a complex mental health disorder that is often accompanied by comorbid disorders. Comorbidity refers to the co-occurrence of two or more disorders in the same individual. The high prevalence of comorbid disorders among people with BPD can make diagnosis and treatment challenging. In this chapter, we will explore some of the common comorbid disorders associated with BPD.

Major Depressive Disorder

Major Depressive Disorder (MDD) is a mood disorder that is characterized by persistent feelings of sadness, hopelessness, and loss of interest in activities. People with BPD are at a higher risk of developing MDD than the general population. The presence of both BPD and MDD can complicate treatment, as both conditions require different treatment approaches.

Anxiety Disorders

Anxiety disorders, such as Generalized Anxiety Disorder (GAD) and Panic Disorder, commonly co-occur with BPD. People with BPD often experience intense fear and anxiety, which can manifest as panic attacks or other anxiety-related symptoms. Anxiety disorders can further exacerbate BPD symptoms and may require specialized treatment.

Substance Use Disorders

Substance use disorders, including alcohol and drug abuse, frequently co-occur with BPD. People with BPD often struggle with impulsive behaviours, which can lead to substance abuse. Substance abuse can further exacerbate BPD symptoms and may require specialized treatment, such as dual diagnosis treatment.

Eating Disorders

Eating disorders, such as Anorexia Nervosa and Bulimia Nervosa, commonly co-occur with BPD. People with BPD often struggle with issues related to self-image, which can lead to disordered eating patterns. Eating disorders can further exacerbate BPD symptoms and may require specialized treatment.

Post-Traumatic Stress Disorder

Post-Traumatic Stress Disorder (PTSD) is a mental health disorder that can develop after exposure to a traumatic event. People with BPD are at a higher risk of developing PTSD than the general population. Both BPD and PTSD involve issues related to emotion regulation, and the presence of both conditions can make treatment more challenging.

Personality Disorders

Other personality disorders, such as Narcissistic Personality Disorder (NPD) and Avoidant Personality Disorder (AvPD), commonly co-occur with BPD. People with BPD often struggle with issues related to self-image and interpersonal relationships, which can lead to the development of other personality disorders.

Attention-Deficit/Hyperactivity Disorder

Attention-Deficit/Hyperactivity Disorder (ADHD) is a neurodevelopmental disorder that is characterized by hyperactivity, impulsivity, and inattention. People with BPD often exhibit symptoms of ADHD, such as impulsivity and difficulty focusing. The presence of both BPD and ADHD can make treatment more challenging.

Conclusion

The high prevalence of comorbid disorders among people with BPD can make diagnosis and treatment challenging. It is essential to identify and treat comorbid disorders in people with BPD to ensure the best possible outcomes. The presence of comorbid disorders can further exacerbate BPD symptoms and may require specialized treatment. By addressing the underlying issues related to both BPD and comorbid disorders, people can learn to manage their symptoms, improve their functioning, and lead more fulfilling lives.

The Role of Genetics in BPD

Borderline Personality Disorder (BPD) is a complex mental health disorder that is believed to be influenced by a combination of environmental and genetic factors. In this chapter, we will explore the role of genetics in BPD.

What are genes?

Genes are segments of DNA that contain the instructions for building and maintaining cells in the body. These instructions determine traits such as eye color, height, and susceptibility to certain diseases. Genes are inherited from both parents, and variations in genes can lead to differences in physical and Behavioural traits.

What is the role of genetics in BPD?

BPD is believed to be a complex disorder with a multifactorial etiology, meaning that it results from the interaction of multiple genetic and environmental factors. Several studies have suggested that genetics play a significant role in the development of BPD. Twin and family studies have shown that BPD has a heritability estimate of around 50 percent, meaning that about half of the variability in BPD symptoms can be attributed to genetic factors.

Several genetic variants have been identified that may be associated with an increased risk of developing BPD. These variants are involved in various processes, such as the regulation of neurotransmitters and the stress response. For example, one study found that a variation in the serotonin transporter gene was associated with an increased risk of BPD.

However, it is important to note that genetic variants associated with BPD are not specific to the disorder and are also found in people without BPD. This suggests that while genetic factors may increase the risk of developing BPD, they do not guarantee the development of the disorder.

Gene-environment interactions in BPD

It is also important to consider the role of gene-environment interactions in the development of BPD. While genetics may increase the risk of developing BPD, environmental factors may also play a crucial role in triggering the onset of the disorder. Childhood trauma, such as abuse or neglect, has been identified as a significant risk factor for BPD. People with a genetic predisposition to BPD may be more vulnerable to the effects of childhood trauma, increasing their risk of developing the disorder.

Research has also suggested that gene-environment interactions may influence the severity and course of BPD. For example, one study found that people with a variation in the oxytocin receptor gene who experienced childhood trauma had more severe BPD symptoms than those without the variation. Another study found that people with a variation in the COMT gene who experienced childhood trauma had a worse response to treatment for BPD.

Conclusion

While genetics play a significant role in the development of BPD, the disorder is believed to result from the interaction of multiple genetic and environmental factors. Identifying specific genetic variants associated with BPD is still an area of active research, and it is important to note that genetic factors are not sufficient to cause the disorder on their own. Gene-environment interactions are crucial to understanding the development, severity, and treatment of BPD. By taking a holistic approach to the assessment and treatment of BPD, including consideration of genetic and environmental factors, individuals with BPD can receive personalized and effective care.

The Emotional Turmoil of BPD

Borderline Personality Disorder (BPD) is often characterized by intense emotional turmoil and instability. In this chapter, we will explore the emotional experiences commonly associated with BPD.

Emotional Dysregulation

Emotional dysregulation is a hallmark of BPD, and it refers to the inability to regulate emotions effectively. People with BPD may experience intense and rapidly shifting emotions, often triggered by seemingly minor events. These emotional fluctuations can be distressing and overwhelming, leading to impulsive behaviours, self-harm, and suicidal thoughts.

Emotional Intensity

People with BPD may experience emotions more intensely than others. They may feel emotions such as anger, sadness, or joy more deeply and for longer periods than others. This intensity can be difficult to manage and can lead to extreme emotional reactions, such as outbursts or self-harm.

Fear of Abandonment

People with BPD often have a profound fear of abandonment, which can drive many of their behaviours and emotions. They may feel intense anxiety and panic at the thought of being alone or rejected, leading to desperate attempts to maintain relationships. This fear of abandonment can also lead to feelings of emptiness and worthlessness.

Self-Image Instability

People with BPD may have a shaky sense of self-identity, which can contribute to emotional instability. They may struggle with feelings of emptiness and an unclear sense of who they are or what they want. This instability can lead to impulsive behaviours, including substance abuse, risky sexual behavior, and self-harm.

Chronic Feelings of Emptiness

Chronic feelings of emptiness are common among people with BPD. They may feel a sense of profound emptiness or numbness, even in the midst of intense emotions. This emptiness can be distressing and may contribute to impulsive behaviours or suicidal thoughts.

Anger and Aggression

People with BPD may experience intense and explosive anger, often triggered by feelings of rejection or abandonment. This anger can lead to aggressive behaviours, including verbal or physical outbursts. These behaviours can be destructive to relationships and can contribute to feelings of shame and guilt.

Guilt and Shame

People with BPD may experience intense feelings of guilt and shame, often related to their impulsive behaviours and emotional reactions. These feelings can be overwhelming and contribute to self-destructive behaviours, such as self-harm or substance abuse. Shame and guilt can also make it difficult for individuals with BPD to seek help or support.

Conclusion

The emotional turmoil experienced by people with BPD can be intense and overwhelming. Emotional dysregulation, fear of abandonment, self-image instability, chronic feelings of emptiness, anger and aggression, and guilt and shame are all common experiences associated with BPD. Understanding and managing these emotions is a crucial component of BPD treatment. Therapies such as Dialectical Behavior Therapy (DBT) focus on developing emotion regulation skills and helping individuals with BPD to tolerate and manage intense emotions. By seeking support and developing coping strategies, individuals with BPD can learn to navigate their emotional experiences and improve their overall well-being.

The Impact of BPD on Personal Relationships

Borderline Personality Disorder (BPD) can have a significant impact on personal relationships. People with BPD may struggle with emotions, interpersonal relationships, and self-identity, making it challenging to maintain stable and healthy relationships. In this chapter, we will explore the impact of BPD on personal relationships.

Difficulty Maintaining Relationships

People with BPD often struggle to maintain stable and healthy relationships. They may experience intense and rapidly shifting emotions that can be overwhelming for their partners. These emotional fluctuations can lead to impulsive behaviours, such as lashing out or self-harm, which can be distressing for partners.

Fear of Abandonment

Fear of abandonment is a common experience for people with BPD, and it can significantly impact their relationships. They may feel intense anxiety and panic at the thought of being rejected or abandoned, leading to desperate attempts to maintain relationships. This fear can lead to clingy or needy behaviours, which can be off-putting for partners and may ultimately strain the relationship.

Idealization and Devaluation

People with BPD may engage in idealization and devaluation of their partners, which can be confusing and distressing for partners. They may put their partners on a pedestal, idealizing them and viewing them as perfect.

However, this idealization can quickly shift to devaluation, where they see their partners as flawed and inadequate. This rapid shift in perception can be jarring for partners and can lead to feelings of confusion and hurt.

Interpersonal Sensitivity

People with BPD may be hypersensitive to interpersonal cues, leading to misinterpretations of their partner's behaviours or intentions. They may perceive slights or criticisms where none were intended, leading to misunderstandings and conflict in relationships. This sensitivity can make it difficult to communicate effectively and can strain relationships.

Chronic Feelings of Emptiness

People with BPD may experience chronic feelings of emptiness, which can contribute to difficulties in relationships. They may struggle to connect with their partners or feel as though they are unable to give or receive love. These feelings can be distressing and may contribute to feelings of isolation and loneliness.

Impulsive Behaviours

People with BPD may engage in impulsive behaviours, which can be damaging to their relationships. They may engage in substance abuse, risky sexual behaviours, or self-harm, which can be distressing and frightening for partners. These behaviours can erode trust in relationships and may lead to feelings of anger and resentment.

Conclusion

BPD can have a significant impact on personal relationships, making it challenging to maintain stable and healthy connections with others. Difficulty maintaining relationships, fear of abandonment, idealization and devaluation, interpersonal sensitivity, chronic feelings of emptiness, and impulsive behaviours are all common experiences associated with BPD that can strain relationships. Seeking treatment and developing coping strategies, such as therapy or support groups, can help individuals with BPD improve their interpersonal relationships and develop healthier, more stable connections with others.

The Challenges of Maintaining Employment with BPD

Borderline Personality Disorder (BPD) can make it challenging to maintain employment. People with BPD may experience intense and rapidly shifting emotions, impulsivity, and difficulties with interpersonal relationships, which can all impact their ability to work. In this chapter, we will explore the challenges of maintaining employment with BPD.

Impulsivity

Impulsivity is a common experience for people with BPD, which can be challenging in the workplace. They may act on impulse, without considering the consequences, leading to poor decision-making or inappropriate behavior. This impulsivity can also lead to difficulties with time management and task completion, which can impact their ability to meet work expectations.

Intense Emotions

People with BPD may experience intense emotions, which can be difficult to manage in the workplace. They may become overwhelmed by their feelings, leading to outbursts or emotional dysregulation, which can be distressing for colleagues and may ultimately impact their ability to perform their job duties.

Interpersonal Difficulties

People with BPD may struggle with interpersonal relationships, which can impact their ability to work effectively with others. They may experience difficulties with communication, misunderstandings, and conflicts with colleagues or superiors. These difficulties can lead to strained relationships, which may ultimately impact their job performance.

Fear of Abandonment

Fear of abandonment is a common experience for people with BPD, which can impact their job stability. They may worry about losing their job or being rejected by their colleagues, leading to anxiety and distress. This fear may also impact their ability to speak up for themselves or assert their needs in the workplace, which can contribute to a sense of powerlessness and dissatisfaction.

Chronic Feelings of Emptiness

People with BPD may experience chronic feelings of emptiness, which can make it difficult to find fulfillment in their work. They may struggle to connect with their colleagues or find meaning in their job duties, leading to a sense of detachment or disengagement. These feelings can impact their motivation and may ultimately impact their job performance.

Treatment Options

Seeking treatment can be helpful for individuals with BPD who are struggling to maintain employment. Therapy, medication, and support groups can all be effective in managing symptoms of BPD and developing coping strategies. Therapy, in particular, can help individuals with BPD develop strategies for managing their emotions, improving interpersonal relationships, and coping with stress in the workplace.

Disclosure and Accommodations

Disclosure of a mental health condition, such as BPD, to an employer can be a difficult decision. However, disclosing may allow for accommodations or support to be provided, such as a flexible work schedule or additional breaks to manage emotions. Some employers may also have an Employee Assistance Program (EAP) that provides counseling services and support to employees with mental health conditions.

Conclusion

Maintaining employment with BPD can be challenging due to difficulties with impulsivity, intense emotions, interpersonal relationships, fear of abandonment, chronic feelings of emptiness, and other symptoms associated with the disorder. Seeking treatment and developing coping strategies can help individuals with BPD manage their symptoms and improve their job performance. Disclosure of the condition and accommodations or support from employers can also be helpful for individuals with BPD who are struggling to maintain employment.

Substance Abuse and BPD

Substance abuse is a common issue among people with Borderline Personality Disorder (BPD). The impulsivity, emotional instability, and low self-esteem that are characteristic of BPD can lead individuals to turn to drugs or alcohol as a way of coping with their symptoms. In this chapter, we will explore the relationship between BPD and substance abuse, and discuss some of the treatment options available for individuals struggling with both.

The Relationship Between BPD and Substance Abuse

Research has shown that there is a high co-occurrence of BPD and substance abuse. One study found that up to 60% of individuals with BPD also have a history of substance abuse or dependence. Another study found that individuals with BPD are more likely to engage in binge drinking and drug use than individuals without the disorder.

The impulsivity and emotional instability associated with BPD can make it difficult for individuals to control their substance use. They may use drugs or alcohol as a way of coping with intense emotions or as a means of self-medicating to alleviate symptoms of BPD. Additionally, individuals with BPD may have difficulty in developing healthy coping strategies, leading them to rely on substance use as a way of managing their symptoms.

The Consequences of Substance Abuse in BPD

Substance abuse can exacerbate the symptoms of BPD, leading to more frequent and intense mood swings, impulsivity, and self-destructive behaviours. It can also interfere with treatment, making it difficult to manage symptoms and achieve stability. Substance abuse can also increase the risk of suicide and self-harm, which are already high in individuals with BPD.

Treatment Options for BPD and Substance Abuse

Treatment for BPD and substance abuse typically involves a combination of therapy and medication. Cognitive-Behavioural therapy (CBT) has been found to be effective in treating both BPD and substance abuse. CBT helps individuals to develop healthy coping strategies, identify triggers for substance use, and develop skills for managing intense emotions.

Dialectical Behavior Therapy (DBT) is another type of therapy that is commonly used to treat BPD. DBT focuses on developing skills for regulating emotions, managing stress, and improving interpersonal relationships. DBT has also been adapted for use in substance abuse treatment, and has been found to be effective in reducing substance use and improving overall functioning.

Medications such as antidepressants and antipsychotics may also be prescribed to treat symptoms of BPD, such as depression and anxiety. Medications may also be prescribed to help manage withdrawal symptoms and cravings associated with substance abuse.

In addition to therapy and medication, support groups can also be beneficial for individuals struggling with both BPD and substance abuse. Support groups provide a safe and non-judgmental environment where individuals can share their experiences and receive support and encouragement from others who are going through similar challenges.

Conclusion

Substance abuse is a common issue among individuals with BPD, due to the impulsivity, emotional instability, and low self-esteem associated with the disorder. Substance abuse can exacerbate symptoms of BPD and interfere with treatment. However, with the right treatment, individuals with BPD and substance abuse can achieve stability and recovery. Therapy, medication, and support groups can all be effective in managing symptoms of both BPD and substance abuse. It is important for individuals with BPD who are struggling with substance abuse to seek professional help and support.

Self-Harm and BPD

Self-harm is a serious concern for people with Borderline Personality Disorder (BPD), with up to 80% of individuals with BPD engaging in self-injurious behaviours at some point in their lives. Self-harm can take various forms, such as cutting, burning, scratching, hitting oneself, or hair-pulling, and it can be an addictive and maladaptive way of coping with intense emotional distress.

Self-harm is often misunderstood and stigmatized, with some people assuming that individuals who engage in self-injury are attention-seeking or suicidal. However, self-harm is usually a way of managing overwhelming emotions, reducing tension, or feeling a sense of control when everything else seems chaotic.

Self-harm behaviours can lead to physical harm, scarring, and infections, and they may also affect the person's social and professional life. Family members and friends of those with BPD may feel scared, helpless, or guilty, as they struggle to understand and address the self-harm.

It's important to remember that self-harm is not a choice, but a manifestation of distress and pain. While it can be challenging to overcome self-harm, it is possible to develop healthier coping strategies and reduce the frequency and severity of self-injurious behaviours. Some effective strategies for dealing with self-harm in BPD include the following:

Identify triggers and warning signs: People with BPD often experience intense emotional dysregulation, such as anger, fear, shame, or abandonment, which can trigger self-harm. Identifying the situations or thoughts that precede self-harm can help to anticipate and prevent it.

Practice self-care: Self-care activities such as exercise, mindfulness, relaxation, or creative hobbies can help to reduce stress and increase self-esteem, making it easier to resist self-harm urges.

Seek professional help: BPD is a complex disorder that requires specialized treatment, and self-harm is often a symptom of an underlying mental health condition. Therapy, medication, or hospitalization may be necessary to manage BPD symptoms and prevent self-harm.

Develop a safety plan: A safety plan is a written strategy that outlines the steps to take when feeling overwhelmed or suicidal. It can include contacting a trusted person, seeking emergency help, or engaging in soothing activities.

Build a support network: People with BPD often feel lonely, misunderstood, or rejected, which can exacerbate self-harm. Building a supportive network of family, friends, or peer groups can provide a sense of belonging and validation.

Challenge negative thoughts and beliefs: Negative thoughts and beliefs, such as "I'm worthless" or "I deserve to be punished," can contribute to self-harm. Learning to identify and challenge these thoughts with more positive and realistic ones can improve self-esteem and reduce self-harm urges.

Explore alternative coping strategies: Instead of self-harm, it's possible to develop healthier coping strategies for managing emotional pain, such as talking to a friend, writing in a journal, listening to music, or using relaxation techniques.

It's essential to remember that recovery from self-harm and BPD is a process that takes time, patience, and support. It's normal to have setbacks and struggles along the way, and seeking professional help can provide the tools and guidance needed to overcome self-harm and improve overall well-being.

Suicidal Ideation and BPD

Suicidal ideation is a common and serious concern for individuals with Borderline Personality Disorder (BPD). In fact, studies have shown that as many as 70% of individuals with BPD have a history of suicidal ideation or attempts. This chapter will explore the complex relationship between suicidal ideation and BPD, and provide information on how individuals with BPD can seek help and support to manage this challenging symptom.

What is Suicidal Ideation?

Suicidal ideation refers to thoughts or ideas about wanting to end one's life. These thoughts can range from fleeting, passing thoughts, to persistent, intense thoughts that consume a person's daily life. Suicidal ideation can be passive (such as thoughts like "I wish I were dead") or active (such as making a plan to end one's life). In some cases, suicidal ideation can be accompanied by suicidal behavior, including attempts to harm oneself or complete suicide.

The Relationship Between BPD and Suicidal Ideation

Individuals with BPD are at a significantly increased risk for suicidal ideation and behavior. This is thought to be due to the intense emotional dysregulation and instability that is a hallmark of the disorder. People with BPD often experience intense feelings of despair, emptiness, and hopelessness, and may struggle to manage these feelings in a healthy way. This can lead to feelings of intense distress, and a desire to escape this distress through suicidal ideation.

In addition to emotional instability, individuals with BPD may also struggle with impulsivity, self-harm, and substance use, all of which increase the risk of suicidal behavior. These individuals may also have a history of trauma, abuse, or neglect, which can further increase the risk of suicidal ideation and behavior.

Managing Suicidal Ideation with BPD

Managing suicidal ideation is a complex and challenging process, and it is important for individuals with BPD to seek professional help and support to manage this symptom. Here are some strategies that may be helpful in managing suicidal ideation with BPD:

Seek Professional Help: If you are experiencing suicidal ideation, it is important to seek professional help as soon as possible. This may involve reaching out to a therapist, counselor, or psychiatrist who specializes in working with individuals with BPD.

Practice Emotional Regulation: One of the most effective ways to manage suicidal ideation is to practice emotional regulation. This may involve learning techniques such as mindfulness, deep breathing, and grounding exercises to help manage intense emotions.

Develop Coping Strategies: It is important to develop coping strategies that can help you manage the intense emotions that can trigger suicidal ideation. This may involve developing a list of activities that you enjoy, such as reading, listening to music, or spending time in nature, that can help distract you from suicidal thoughts.

Connect with Others: Social support is an important factor in managing suicidal ideation. This may involve reaching out to friends, family members, or support groups for help and support.

Create a Safety Plan: It is important to create a safety plan that outlines what steps you will take if you experience suicidal ideation. This may involve identifying warning signs, developing a list of emergency contacts, and creating a plan for what to do if you experience a crisis.

Conclusion

Suicidal ideation is a serious concern for individuals with Borderline Personality Disorder. However, with the right support and management strategies, it is possible to manage this challenging symptom. If you or someone you know is experiencing suicidal ideation, it is important to seek professional help as soon as possible. Remember that help is available, and that you do not have to face this challenge alone.

Treatment Options for BPD

Borderline Personality Disorder (BPD) is a complex and challenging condition to manage. It requires a comprehensive treatment plan that may involve multiple forms of therapy and medication. The goal of treatment is to help individuals with BPD learn how to regulate their emotions and reduce impulsivity, improve interpersonal relationships, and enhance their overall quality of life.

There are several treatment options available for individuals with BPD. The following are some of the most common forms of treatment for BPD.

Psychotherapy: Psychotherapy, or talk therapy, is often the first line of treatment for individuals with BPD. Different types of psychotherapy have been shown to be effective in treating BPD. Some of the most commonly used psychotherapies include:

Dialectical Behavior Therapy (DBT): DBT is a form of cognitive-Behavioural therapy that was developed specifically to treat BPD. DBT teaches skills for emotion regulation, distress tolerance, interpersonal effectiveness, and mindfulness.

Cognitive Behavioural Therapy (CBT): CBT focuses on identifying and changing negative patterns of thinking and behavior. CBT can be effective in treating symptoms of depression and anxiety that often co-occur with BPD.

Schema Therapy: Schema Therapy is a form of psychotherapy that focuses on changing negative patterns of thinking and behavior that developed in childhood. It can be effective in treating BPD symptoms related to attachment and abandonment issues.

Medication: There are no medications specifically approved for the treatment of BPD. However, some medications may be used to treat specific symptoms, such as mood swings, anxiety, and depression. Some commonly used medications include:

Antidepressants: Antidepressants are often used to treat symptoms of depression and anxiety that co-occur with BPD.

Mood Stabilizers: Mood stabilizers, such as lithium, can help reduce mood swings and impulsivity.

Antipsychotics: Antipsychotics are sometimes used to treat symptoms of psychosis, such as hallucinations and delusions.

Group Therapy: Group therapy can be an effective form of treatment for individuals with BPD. Group therapy provides an opportunity for individuals to practice interpersonal skills and receive support from others who are going through similar experiences.

Family Therapy: Family therapy can be helpful in treating BPD, as it can help improve communication and reduce conflict within the family.

Mindfulness-Based Interventions: Mindfulness-based interventions, such as meditation and yoga, can help individuals with BPD learn how to regulate their emotions and reduce stress.

It is important to note that treatment for BPD often involves a combination of therapies. For example, a person with BPD may receive DBT and medication, as well as participate in group therapy.

In addition to these treatment options, there are also several self-help strategies that can be effective in managing BPD symptoms. These include:

Self-Care: Engaging in self-care activities, such as exercise, getting enough sleep, and eating a healthy diet, can help improve overall well-being and reduce stress.

Journaling: Keeping a journal can be an effective way to process emotions and identify patterns of thinking and behavior.

Mindfulness: Practicing mindfulness can help individuals with BPD learn how to regulate their emotions and reduce impulsivity.

Building Support Systems: Building a support system of family, friends, and mental health professionals can provide individuals with BPD with the emotional support they need to manage their symptoms.

Overall, BPD is a challenging condition to manage, but with the right treatment and support, individuals with BPD can learn how to regulate their emotions, improve their relationships, and enhance their overall quality of life.

Psychotherapy Approaches for BPD

Psychotherapy, or talk therapy, is a crucial aspect of treating borderline personality disorder (BPD). It can help individuals with BPD gain insight into their thoughts and behaviours, learn coping strategies, and improve their relationships. There are several different approaches to psychotherapy that may be used to treat BPD, each with its own strengths and limitations.

Dialectical Behavior Therapy (DBT)

DBT is a type of cognitive-Behavioural therapy that was developed specifically for the treatment of BPD. It focuses on four core areas: mindfulness, distress tolerance, emotion regulation, and interpersonal effectiveness. DBT helps individuals with BPD learn to identify and regulate their emotions, cope with distressing situations, and improve their communication skills.

Cognitive-Behavioural Therapy (CBT)

CBT is a type of therapy that focuses on changing negative patterns of thought and behavior. It is often used to treat a variety of mental health conditions, including BPD. CBT for BPD typically focuses on identifying and challenging maladaptive beliefs, developing coping skills, and improving communication skills.

Psychodynamic Therapy

Psychodynamic therapy is a form of talk therapy that focuses on exploring unconscious thoughts and feelings that may be contributing to a person's mental health concerns. It can be used to treat BPD by helping individuals gain insight into their relationships and behaviours.

Mentalization-Based Therapy (MBT)

MBT is a form of psychotherapy that focuses on improving a person's ability to understand their own thoughts and feelings, as well as the thoughts and feelings of others. It can be particularly helpful for individuals with BPD who struggle with interpersonal relationships.

Schema-Focused Therapy

Schema-focused therapy is a type of psychotherapy that focuses on identifying and changing deeply ingrained patterns of thought and behavior, called schemas. It can be used to treat BPD by helping individuals identify and challenge maladaptive schemas, and develop more adaptive coping strategies.

Transference-Focused Therapy (TFT)

TFT is a form of psychodynamic therapy that focuses on exploring the ways in which a person's past experiences and relationships may be affecting their current relationships and behaviours. It can be particularly helpful for individuals with BPD who struggle with interpersonal relationships.

Group Therapy

Group therapy can be a helpful addition to individual psychotherapy for individuals with BPD. It provides a supportive environment in which individuals can practice their communication and interpersonal skills, receive feedback from others, and develop a sense of community.

Family Therapy

Family therapy can be helpful for individuals with BPD whose family members are also involved in therapy. It can help families learn to communicate more effectively, set boundaries, and work together to support the individual with BPD.

Overall, psychotherapy is an important component of treating BPD. It can help individuals learn to manage their emotions, improve their relationships, and develop a more positive sense of self. The specific approach to psychotherapy will depend on the individual's unique needs and preferences, as well as the therapist's expertise and training. It is important to work with a mental health professional who has experience treating BPD and who can tailor treatment to your specific needs.

Medication Treatment for BPD

Borderline personality disorder (BPD) is a complex mental health condition that can be challenging to treat. Psychotherapy is considered the first-line treatment for BPD. However, medication can also be helpful in managing symptoms and improving the quality of life for people with BPD. In this chapter, we will explore medication treatment options for BPD.

Medication treatment for BPD is often used in conjunction with psychotherapy. Medication alone is not sufficient to treat BPD, but it can help manage symptoms such as mood swings, anxiety, and depression. The following are some of the medication options available for treating BPD.

Antidepressants: Antidepressants are commonly prescribed for BPD, even if the person does not have depression. Antidepressants can help stabilize mood, reduce anxiety, and improve sleep. Selective serotonin reuptake inhibitors (SSRIs) and serotonin-norepinephrine reuptake inhibitors (SNRIs) are the most commonly prescribed antidepressants for BPD.

Mood stabilizers: Mood stabilizers, such as lithium and valproate, can be used to manage mood swings and impulsive behavior in people with BPD. These medications are often prescribed for bipolar disorder, but they can also be effective in treating BPD.

Antipsychotics: Antipsychotic medications, such as risperidone and olanzapine, can help manage symptoms of psychosis, such as delusions and hallucinations. They can also help stabilize mood and reduce impulsive behavior.

Anti-anxiety medications: Anti-anxiety medications, such as benzodiazepines, can be helpful in reducing anxiety and agitation. However, they should be used with caution as they can be addictive and can lead to dependence.

Stimulants: Stimulant medications, such as methylphenidate, can be used to improve attention and concentration in people with BPD who also have attention deficit hyperactivity disorder (ADHD).

It is important to note that medication treatment for BPD is not a one-size-fits-all approach. The choice of medication depends on the individual's symptoms and the severity of their BPD. Additionally, medication treatment for BPD should be closely monitored by a healthcare professional to ensure that the person is responding well to the medication and is not experiencing any adverse side effects.

It is also essential to understand that medication treatment for BPD is not a cure. Medication can help manage symptoms, but it does not address the underlying causes of BPD. Therefore, medication treatment should be used in conjunction with psychotherapy to provide a comprehensive approach to treating BPD.

In some cases, medication may be prescribed for a limited period, such as during a crisis, to help manage severe symptoms. In other cases, medication may be prescribed for a longer period to help manage chronic symptoms. The duration of medication treatment should be determined by the person's healthcare provider.

It is also essential to understand that medication treatment for BPD may not work for everyone. Some people may not respond well to medication, while others may experience adverse side effects. If a person does not respond well to medication, their healthcare provider may need to adjust the dosage or switch to a different medication.

In conclusion, medication treatment can be a helpful tool in managing symptoms of BPD, such as mood swings, anxiety, and depression. However, medication treatment should be used in conjunction with psychotherapy to provide a comprehensive approach to treating BPD. The choice of medication depends on the individual's symptoms and the severity of their BPD, and medication treatment should be closely monitored by a healthcare professional to ensure that the person is responding well to the medication and is not experiencing any adverse side effects.

Alternative and Complementary Therapies for BPD

Borderline personality disorder (BPD) is a complex mental health condition that can cause significant distress and impairment in daily life. While psychotherapy and medication are the primary treatments for BPD, some individuals may benefit from alternative and complementary therapies as well. In this chapter, we will explore some of the options available for those seeking additional forms of treatment for BPD.

Dialectical Behavior Therapy (DBT)

DBT is a form of psychotherapy specifically developed for individuals with BPD. This therapy combines cognitive-Behavioural techniques with mindfulness practices to help individuals manage their emotions, improve their relationships, and reduce self-destructive behaviours. DBT typically involves weekly individual therapy sessions, group therapy sessions, and homework assignments.

Eye Movement Desensitization and Reprocessing (EMDR)

EMDR is a psychotherapy approach that has been used to treat various mental health conditions, including BPD. This therapy involves guided eye movements or other forms of bilateral stimulation while the individual recalls distressing memories or experiences. The goal of EMDR is to help the individual process and resolve these traumatic experiences.

Acceptance and Commitment Therapy (ACT)

ACT is a type of psychotherapy that helps individuals develop psychological flexibility and acceptance of their emotions and experiences. This therapy involves mindfulness practices, values clarification, and commitment to taking action towards one's goals.

Mindfulness-Based Stress Reduction (MBSR)

MBSR is a mindfulness-based program that has been used to treat various mental health conditions, including BPD. This program involves guided meditations, body scans, and other mindfulness practices to help individuals manage stress and improve their overall well-being.

Art Therapy

Art therapy is a form of psychotherapy that involves the use of art materials and creative expression to help individuals explore their emotions and experiences. This therapy can be particularly useful for individuals who have difficulty expressing themselves verbally.

Yoga

Yoga is a mind-body practice that has been shown to have numerous benefits for mental health, including reducing anxiety and depression. Some individuals with BPD may find that regular yoga practice helps them manage their emotions and improve their overall well-being.

Acupuncture

Acupuncture is a form of traditional Chinese medicine that involves the insertion of thin needles into specific points on the body. Some individuals with BPD may find that acupuncture helps reduce anxiety, improve sleep, and promote overall relaxation.

Massage Therapy

Massage therapy is a form of bodywork that involves the manipulation of muscles and soft tissues. This therapy can be particularly useful for individuals who experience physical tension as a result of their emotional distress.

Nutrition and Supplementation

While there is no specific diet or supplement that can cure BPD, some individuals may find that certain dietary changes or supplements can help improve their overall well-being. For example, omega-3 fatty acids have been shown to have anti-inflammatory properties and may help reduce symptoms of depression and anxiety.

Essential Oils

Essential oils are concentrated plant extracts that are used in aromatherapy. Some essential oils, such as lavender and chamomile, have been shown to have calming effects and may help reduce anxiety and promote relaxation.

It is important to note that while these alternative and complementary therapies may be helpful for some individuals with BPD, they should not be used as a substitute for evidence-based treatments such as psychotherapy and medication. It is also essential to work with a qualified healthcare provider to determine the most appropriate treatment plan for your specific needs.

Self-Help Strategies for Managing BPD Symptoms

Borderline Personality Disorder (BPD) is a complex mental health condition that can greatly impact an individual's daily life. While professional treatment is often necessary for managing BPD symptoms, there are also self-help strategies that can be helpful for individuals with BPD to manage their symptoms and improve their overall well-being.

Educate Yourself: Knowledge is power, and it can be empowering to learn more about BPD and the specific symptoms you experience. This can help you understand your behavior and emotions better and allow you to develop more effective coping mechanisms.

Develop a Support System: It can be helpful to have people in your life who understand and support you. Consider joining a support group, connecting with others with BPD, or reaching out to family and friends.

Practice Mindfulness: Mindfulness is a technique that involves being present and non-judgmental in the moment. Practicing mindfulness can help individuals with BPD better manage their emotions and regulate their mood.

Engage in Regular Exercise: Exercise is a great way to reduce stress, improve mood, and increase feelings of well-being. Regular exercise can be a helpful tool in managing BPD symptoms.

Get Enough Sleep: Sleep is critical for both physical and mental health. Aim to get at least 7-8 hours of sleep each night, and develop a consistent sleep routine.

Practice Self-Care: Engage in activities that make you feel good and promote well-being. This can include things like taking a warm bath, reading a book, or engaging in a hobby.

Set Realistic Goals: Setting goals that are achievable can help you feel more confident and in control. Start small and work towards larger goals over time.

Develop Coping Strategies: Identify coping strategies that work well for you and practice using them regularly. This can include techniques like deep breathing, positive self-talk, or progressive muscle relaxation.

Avoid Substance Abuse: Substance abuse can exacerbate BPD symptoms and make it more difficult to manage. Avoid drugs and alcohol, and seek professional help if you are struggling with addiction.

Stay Engaged with Treatment: It's important to stay engaged with professional treatment even when you are feeling better. Attend therapy sessions regularly and take any medications as prescribed.

Manage Stress: Stress can trigger BPD symptoms, so it's important to manage stress effectively. This can include techniques like meditation, deep breathing, or exercise.

Set Boundaries: Setting boundaries in relationships can help you manage your emotions and reduce stress. Practice saying "no" when you need to, and communicate your needs to others.

Learn to Validate Yourself: Validation is the process of recognizing and accepting your emotions. Learning to validate yourself can help you manage your emotions more effectively and reduce feelings of distress.

Practice Gratitude: Practicing gratitude can help you focus on the positive aspects of your life and increase feelings of well-being. Take time each day to reflect on what you are grateful for.

Challenge Negative Thoughts: Negative thoughts can exacerbate BPD symptoms. Practice challenging negative thoughts and replacing them with more positive, realistic thoughts.

Develop a Crisis Plan: It can be helpful to have a crisis plan in place in case of a mental health emergency. This can include a list of emergency contacts, coping strategies, and professional resources.

Practice Forgiveness: Forgiveness can help reduce feelings of anger and resentment, which are common in individuals with BPD. Practice forgiving yourself and others to promote emotional healing.

Express Yourself Creatively: Engage in creative activities, like painting or writing, to help process emotions and promote well-being.

Mindfulness Techniques for BPD

Mindfulness techniques are effective in reducing the symptoms of borderline personality disorder (BPD). These techniques can help BPD patients to manage their emotions and thoughts, and promote a more balanced and stable mindset. In this chapter, we will explore mindfulness techniques that can be helpful in managing BPD symptoms.

What is Mindfulness?

Mindfulness is a meditation practice that involves paying attention to the present moment without judgment. It is about focusing on the here and now, rather than worrying about the past or future. Mindfulness helps to increase awareness, reduce stress, and improve mental health.

Mindfulness-Based Cognitive Therapy (MBCT)

MBCT is an evidence-based therapy that combines mindfulness meditation and cognitive-Behavioural therapy (CBT). It is a group-based program that teaches mindfulness techniques to help individuals manage their emotions and thoughts. MBCT has been shown to be effective in reducing the symptoms of depression, anxiety, and stress, which are common comorbidities of BPD.

Body Scan

The body scan technique involves focusing on each part of the body, from the toes to the head, and observing any sensations or feelings without judgment. This technique can help individuals to become more aware of their physical sensations and improve their mind-body connection.

Practicing the body scan technique regularly can help BPD patients to become more grounded and centered.

Breathing Meditation

Breathing meditation involves paying attention to the breath and observing any sensations without judgment. This technique helps to calm the mind and reduce stress. BPD patients can practice breathing meditation anytime and anywhere, such as during a stressful situation or before going to bed. By focusing on the breath, individuals can gain a sense of control and calmness.

Mindful Eating

Mindful eating is about paying attention to the experience of eating, such as the smell, taste, and texture of food. It involves eating slowly and savoring each bite, rather than rushing through a meal. This technique can help BPD patients to develop a healthier relationship with food, reduce emotional eating, and promote mindful awareness in daily life.

Mindful Walking

Mindful walking is a technique that involves focusing on the sensations of walking, such as the movement of the legs and the feeling of the feet on the ground. It is a form of walking meditation that can help individuals to become more present and mindful. BPD patients can practice mindful walking during a walk in the park or while doing errands. This technique can help to reduce stress and promote a sense of calmness.

Journaling

Journaling is a mindfulness technique that involves writing down thoughts and feelings without judgment. It can help BPD patients to express themselves and gain insight into their emotions and thoughts. By becoming more aware of their emotions, individuals can learn to manage them more effectively.

Conclusion

Mindfulness techniques can be an effective tool for managing the symptoms of BPD. By practicing mindfulness regularly, individuals can become more aware of their emotions and thoughts, and develop a more balanced and stable mindset. Mindfulness-based therapies such as MBCT, body scan, breathing meditation, mindful eating, mindful walking, and journaling are all helpful techniques that can be incorporated into a BPD treatment plan. With commitment and practice, individuals can learn to manage their BPD symptoms and improve their overall quality of life.

Dialectical Behaviour Therapy (DBT) for BPD

Dialectical Behaviour Therapy (DBT) is a form of cognitive behavioural therapy that is specifically designed to treat individuals with borderline personality disorder (BPD). DBT combines individual therapy, group skills training, phone coaching, and consultation for the therapist. It was developed in the 1980s by Dr. Marsha Linehan, who found that traditional CBT approaches were not effective for individuals with BPD due to their difficulty regulating their emotions.

DBT is based on the concept of dialectics, which is the idea that two opposing ideas can be true at the same time. In the case of BPD, this means accepting the individual as they are while also acknowledging that they need to change some of their behaviours to live a fulfilling life. DBT focuses on four main areas: mindfulness, distress tolerance, emotion regulation, and interpersonal effectiveness.

Mindfulness involves learning to be present in the moment without judgment. This is particularly important for individuals with BPD who may struggle with intense emotions that can take over their thoughts and behaviours. By practicing mindfulness, individuals can learn to observe their emotions without becoming overwhelmed by them.

Distress tolerance is another key component of DBT. This involves learning to tolerate difficult emotions without engaging in harmful behaviours, such as self-harm or substance abuse. Individuals learn coping strategies such as distraction, self-soothing, and mindfulness to help them manage distressing emotions.

Emotion regulation is focused on helping individuals learn to identify and understand their emotions, as well as develop strategies to manage intense emotions. This can include techniques such as changing negative thoughts, increasing positive experiences, and problem-solving skills.

Finally, interpersonal effectiveness focuses on teaching individuals skills to improve their communication and relationships with others. This includes assertiveness training, conflict resolution, and learning to set boundaries.

DBT is typically delivered in a structured program that includes individual therapy, group skills training, and phone coaching. In individual therapy, the therapist works with the individual to develop skills to manage their emotions and improve their relationships. Group skills training is focused on teaching specific skills related to mindfulness, distress tolerance, emotion regulation, and interpersonal effectiveness. Phone coaching is provided to help individuals apply their new skills in real-world situations.

Research has shown that DBT is an effective treatment for BPD. Studies have found that individuals who receive DBT experience a significant reduction in suicidal behaviour, self-harm, and hospitalization. Additionally, individuals who receive DBT have shown improvements in their ability to regulate their emotions, manage stress, and maintain relationships.

DBT has also been found to be effective for treating other mental health disorders, such as depression, anxiety, and substance use disorders. This is because the skills taught in DBT are applicable to a wide range of emotional and behavioural issues.

In conclusion, Dialectical Behaviour Therapy (DBT) is a highly effective treatment option for individuals with borderline personality disorder. DBT focuses on developing skills in mindfulness, distress tolerance, emotion regulation, and interpersonal effectiveness. By teaching individuals to manage their emotions and improve their relationships, DBT has been shown to significantly reduce suicidal behaviour, self-harm, and hospitalization. If you or someone you know is struggling with BPD, DBT may be a valuable treatment option to consider.

Cognitive Behavioural Therapy (CBT) for BPD

Cognitive Behavioural Therapy (CBT) is a widely recognized form of psychotherapy that is often used to treat various mental health disorders, including borderline personality disorder (BPD). CBT focuses on identifying and changing negative thought patterns and behaviours to improve mental health and overall well-being. In this chapter, we will explore the use of CBT in treating BPD and its effectiveness.

CBT is based on the premise that our thoughts, feelings, and behaviours are interconnected. It suggests that the way we think about a situation affects how we feel and behave. Therefore, by changing negative thoughts into more positive ones, we can change our feelings and behaviours accordingly.

In the case of BPD, individuals often experience intense and unstable emotions, have negative self-images, and engage in impulsive and self-destructive behaviours. CBT can help individuals with BPD identify and challenge negative thoughts and beliefs that contribute to these symptoms. By doing so, they can develop new coping strategies and problem-solving skills to better manage their emotions and behaviours.

One of the primary techniques used in CBT is cognitive restructuring. Cognitive restructuring involves identifying negative thoughts and beliefs and replacing them with more positive and realistic ones. For example, an individual with BPD may have negative thoughts about themselves such as “I am a failure,” or “I am unlovable.” These thoughts may contribute to feelings of sadness, hopelessness, and low self-esteem, which can in turn lead to impulsive and self-destructive behaviours.

Through cognitive restructuring, individuals can learn to challenge these negative thoughts and replace them with more realistic and positive ones such as “I am not perfect, but I am capable of learning and growing,” or “I am worthy of love and respect.” By doing so, they can improve their self-esteem, reduce their negative emotions, and reduce the likelihood of engaging in self-destructive behaviours.

Another technique used in CBT is Behavioural activation. Behavioural activation involves identifying and engaging in activities that bring joy and a sense of accomplishment. This technique can be particularly helpful for individuals with BPD who may struggle with low motivation and feelings of emptiness. By engaging in activities that are meaningful and rewarding, individuals can improve their mood and sense of purpose.

CBT for BPD often includes elements of mindfulness-based therapy, which involves developing a non-judgmental awareness of the present moment. Mindfulness can help individuals with BPD learn to observe their emotions without judgment or reaction, which can help reduce their intensity and frequency. Mindfulness can also help individuals with BPD learn to tolerate distressing emotions, which is a crucial skill for managing their symptoms.

CBT has been shown to be an effective treatment for BPD, particularly when combined with other forms of therapy, such as DBT. A meta-analysis of 19 studies found that CBT was associated with significant improvements in BPD symptoms, including reduced self-harm behaviours, reduced depression, and improved social functioning (Stoffers et al., 2012). However, like all forms of therapy, CBT may not be effective for everyone, and individuals may need to try different forms of therapy to find what works best for them.

In summary, CBT is a form of psychotherapy that can be used to treat BPD. It focuses on identifying and changing negative thoughts and behaviours to improve mental health and overall well-being. CBT techniques such as cognitive restructuring, Behavioural activation, and mindfulness-based therapy can help individuals with BPD improve their emotional regulation, reduce their negative emotions, and reduce the likelihood of engaging in self-destructive behaviours. While CBT has been shown to be effective in treating BPD, it may not work for everyone, and individuals may need to try different forms of therapy to find what works best for them.

Psychodynamic Therapy for BPD

Psychodynamic therapy is a form of psychotherapy that aims to help individuals identify and resolve their unconscious conflicts and unresolved emotional issues that may be contributing to their current psychological distress. This therapeutic approach can be useful in treating individuals with borderline personality disorder (BPD), who often have a history of unresolved emotional traumas and interpersonal difficulties.

The psychodynamic approach to BPD treatment involves exploring the underlying causes of the individual's symptoms and behavior patterns. The therapist aims to develop a trusting and supportive relationship with the client, which enables the client to explore their emotions and experiences in a safe and non-judgmental environment.

One of the primary goals of psychodynamic therapy for BPD is to help the individual develop a sense of self-awareness. This involves exploring the individual's sense of self, their beliefs and values, and their emotional responses to different situations. The therapist can help the individual identify any self-destructive patterns or behaviours that may be causing them harm and help them develop healthier coping mechanisms.

Another key component of psychodynamic therapy for BPD is exploring the individual's relationship patterns. BPD is often characterized by unstable and intense interpersonal relationships, which can be difficult to manage. By exploring the individual's past relationships, the therapist can help them identify any unhealthy patterns and work towards developing healthier relationships in the future.

Psychodynamic therapy can also help individuals with BPD address their feelings of abandonment and rejection. BPD is often associated with a fear of abandonment, which can lead to intense emotional responses and unstable relationships. Through therapy, the individual can explore their feelings of abandonment and develop coping mechanisms to manage these feelings.

Overall, psychodynamic therapy can be an effective treatment option for individuals with BPD. It can help individuals gain insight into their emotional patterns and develop healthier coping mechanisms to manage their symptoms. However, it is important to note that this type of therapy can be a long-term process and may not be suitable for everyone. It is important to work with a therapist who specializes in psychodynamic therapy and has experience working with individuals with BPD.

Interpersonal Therapy for BPD

Interpersonal therapy (IPT) is a time-limited, evidence-based therapy that focuses on the interpersonal relationships and communication patterns of individuals with borderline personality disorder (BPD). It aims to improve the quality of these relationships and communication patterns, which in turn leads to improved mood and reduced symptoms.

IPT was initially developed for the treatment of depression, but has since been adapted and applied to other mental health disorders, including BPD. IPT typically involves 12-16 weekly sessions, with each session lasting approximately one hour.

The goal of IPT for BPD is to help individuals develop more effective communication and interpersonal skills. This includes learning how to express their needs and emotions more clearly, how to identify and address interpersonal problems, and how to develop more fulfilling relationships with others.

IPT for BPD typically focuses on four interpersonal problem areas:

Grief: This involves helping individuals process and cope with losses, such as the end of a relationship or the death of a loved one.

Role transitions: This involves helping individuals adjust to significant changes in their lives, such as starting a new job or becoming a parent.

Interpersonal disputes: This involves helping individuals resolve conflicts with others in a constructive and respectful manner.

Interpersonal deficits: This involves helping individuals develop and improve their communication and interpersonal skills, such as assertiveness, empathy, and active listening.

IPT for BPD typically begins with an assessment phase, during which the therapist and client work together to identify the interpersonal problem areas that are most relevant to the individual's current situation. The therapist then helps the client develop specific goals and strategies for addressing these problem areas.

One of the key techniques used in IPT for BPD is role-playing, in which the therapist and client act out different scenarios and communication patterns to help the client develop more effective interpersonal skills. The therapist may also assign homework assignments, such as practicing specific communication skills with family members or friends.

Several studies have found that IPT can be an effective treatment for BPD, particularly when used in combination with other therapies, such as DBT or medication. For example, a randomized controlled trial found that IPT was as effective as DBT in reducing BPD symptoms and improving interpersonal functioning, and that the two therapies had complementary effects.

Overall, IPT is a promising treatment option for individuals with BPD who struggle with interpersonal problems and communication difficulties. However, as with any therapy, it is important to work with a qualified therapist who has experience in treating BPD and who can tailor the treatment approach to meet your specific needs and goals.

Group Therapy for BPD

Group therapy is a popular form of treatment for individuals with borderline personality disorder (BPD). It provides a supportive environment where individuals can share their experiences with others who have similar struggles. This chapter will discuss group therapy as a treatment option for BPD, including its benefits and how it works.

Group therapy for BPD typically involves a group of six to twelve individuals with BPD who meet regularly with a trained therapist. The therapy can take many forms, including psychoeducational groups, skills groups, and process-oriented groups. Each type of group therapy has its own focus, but all aim to provide participants with tools and support to manage their BPD symptoms.

Psychoeducational groups are focused on teaching participants about BPD and how it affects their thoughts, feelings, and behaviours. Participants learn about the symptoms of BPD, as well as coping strategies and treatment options. These groups are often structured and provide participants with a set curriculum.

Skills groups are focused on teaching participants specific skills to manage their BPD symptoms. These may include mindfulness meditation, emotion regulation techniques, interpersonal effectiveness, and distress tolerance. Participants learn these skills through experiential exercises and homework assignments.

Process-oriented groups are focused on helping participants explore and understand their thoughts, feelings, and behaviours in the context of their relationships with others. Participants are encouraged to share their experiences and support each other through the therapeutic process.

One of the primary benefits of group therapy for BPD is the opportunity to connect with others who have similar struggles. Individuals with BPD often feel isolated and misunderstood, and group therapy can provide a sense of belonging and validation. Participants can also learn from each other's experiences and offer support and encouragement.

Group therapy can also be more cost-effective than individual therapy, as the therapist's time and resources are shared among multiple participants. This can make it a more accessible option for individuals who may not be able to afford individual therapy.

Another benefit of group therapy is the opportunity to practice interpersonal skills in a safe and supportive environment. Many individuals with BPD struggle with interpersonal relationships, and group therapy can provide a space to practice communication, boundaries, and conflict resolution.

Group therapy for BPD is often structured and goal-oriented, with a clear focus on symptom management and skill-building. Participants are encouraged to set goals and work towards them with the support of the therapist and other group members. This can provide a sense of empowerment and progress, which can be motivating for individuals with BPD.

Group therapy is not without its challenges, however. Some individuals may feel uncomfortable sharing their experiences with others, or may struggle with social anxiety. It is important for the therapist to create a safe and supportive environment and to be sensitive to individual needs and preferences.

In addition, group therapy is not appropriate for everyone with BPD. Individuals with severe symptoms or who are at high risk for suicide may require more intensive individual treatment before participating in a group.

Overall, group therapy can be an effective treatment option for individuals with BPD. It provides a supportive environment where individuals can learn new skills and connect with others who have similar struggles. If you are considering group therapy for BPD, it is important to find a qualified therapist with experience in treating BPD and to carefully consider whether it is the right treatment option for you.

Family Therapy for BPD

Family therapy is a form of psychotherapy that focuses on improving communication and relationships among family members. It has been found to be effective in treating a wide range of mental health conditions, including borderline personality disorder (BPD). Family therapy for BPD can help family members better understand the disorder and learn how to support their loved one with the condition.

The goal of family therapy for BPD is to improve communication and increase understanding between family members. This can be especially important in families where there is a history of conflict or where there is a lack of understanding about BPD. Family therapy can help family members learn new skills and strategies for interacting with their loved one with BPD in a more positive and supportive way.

Family therapy typically involves a series of sessions with a trained therapist. During these sessions, the therapist will work with the family to identify the specific challenges they are facing and to develop strategies for addressing them. The therapist may use a variety of techniques, such as role-playing, communication exercises, and education about BPD.

One of the key components of family therapy for BPD is psychoeducation. This involves educating family members about the symptoms and causes of BPD, as well as the treatment options that are available. By understanding the disorder more fully, family members are better able to provide support and to avoid behaviours that may exacerbate symptoms.

Another important aspect of family therapy for BPD is learning how to communicate more effectively. Many people with BPD struggle with communication, which can lead to misunderstandings and conflict with loved ones. Family therapy can help family members learn how to communicate in a way that is more supportive and less confrontational.

In addition to improving communication, family therapy for BPD can also help family members learn how to set healthy boundaries. People with BPD often struggle with boundaries, which can lead to unstable relationships and feelings of rejection or abandonment. Family therapy can help family members learn how to set and maintain boundaries that are respectful and supportive.

Family therapy can also help family members learn how to manage their own emotions in response to their loved one's BPD. Many family members of people with BPD experience stress, anxiety, and other negative emotions as a result of their loved one's condition. Family therapy can help family members learn how to manage these emotions in a healthy way and to avoid behaviours that may exacerbate their loved one's symptoms.

Finally, family therapy can help family members develop a plan for ongoing support and care for their loved one with BPD. This may include identifying additional resources and support networks, developing a crisis plan for emergencies, and setting goals for ongoing treatment and recovery.

Overall, family therapy can be an effective treatment option for people with BPD and their loved ones. By improving communication, setting healthy boundaries, and providing ongoing support, family therapy can help people with BPD and their families learn to manage the challenges of the disorder and to build more stable and supportive relationships.

The Importance of a Support System for BPD Recovery

Borderline personality disorder (BPD) can be a challenging condition to manage, but with the right support system, recovery is possible. Having a strong support system is crucial for those with BPD as it helps to reduce feelings of isolation, provides emotional and practical support, and helps individuals stay motivated and committed to their treatment. In this chapter, we will discuss the importance of a support system for BPD recovery.

What is a support system?

A support system can be defined as a group of people who provide emotional, practical, and sometimes financial support to an individual who is going through a difficult time. Support systems can be made up of family, friends, mental health professionals, support groups, and other community resources. For individuals with BPD, a support system can be an essential part of their recovery journey.

The benefits of a support system

Having a strong support system can have a significant impact on a person's mental health and well-being. Below are some of the benefits of having a support system for those with BPD:

Reduces feelings of isolation: Individuals with BPD often feel alone and isolated. Having a support system can help them feel connected to others and reduce their feelings of loneliness.

Provides emotional support: Living with BPD can be emotionally taxing. Having a support system can provide a safe space to share thoughts and feelings and receive emotional support.

Provides practical support: A support system can provide practical help with daily tasks, such as grocery shopping, cooking, and cleaning. This practical support can help individuals with BPD manage their symptoms and focus on their recovery.

Helps to stay motivated: Recovery from BPD can be a long and challenging journey. Having a support system can help individuals stay motivated and committed to their treatment.

Improves self-esteem: Being part of a support system can help individuals with BPD feel valued and appreciated, which can boost their self-esteem.

Types of support systems for BPD

There are several types of support systems that individuals with BPD can utilize. These include:

Family and friends: Loved ones can be an essential source of support for individuals with BPD. They can offer emotional and practical support and provide a sense of security and stability.

Mental health professionals: Mental health professionals, such as therapists, psychiatrists, and social workers, can provide therapy and medication management to help manage symptoms of BPD.

Support groups: Joining a support group can be a great way to connect with others who are going through similar experiences. Support groups can provide a sense of community, emotional support, and practical advice.

Community resources: Community resources, such as crisis hotlines, shelters, and community mental health clinics, can provide additional support for individuals with BPD.

Tips for building a support system

Building a support system can take time and effort, but it is worth it. Below are some tips for building a support system for BPD recovery:

Reach out to loved ones: Let your family and friends know that you need their support. Be honest about your struggles and ask for help when you need it.

Find a mental health professional: A mental health professional can provide individual therapy and medication management. They can also help connect you to other resources, such as support groups.

Join a support group: Look for support groups in your community or online. Joining a support group can provide emotional support and practical advice.

Utilize community resources: There are several community resources available for individuals with BPD. Crisis hotlines, shelters, and community mental health clinics can provide additional support.

Borderline Personality Disorder (BPD) not only affects the individual diagnosed with the disorder but also has a significant impact on the lives of their family members. Family members of someone with BPD often find themselves in a difficult situation, struggling to understand their loved one's behavior and cope with the emotional toll the disorder can take on them. In this chapter, we will discuss coping strategies that family members of someone with BPD can use to manage their own emotions and support their loved one's recovery.

Educate Yourself About BPD

One of the most important things family members can do is to educate themselves about BPD. This includes understanding the symptoms of the disorder, how it is diagnosed, and the treatment options available. It can be helpful to attend therapy sessions with your loved one and participate in family therapy to gain a better understanding of the disorder and learn how to support your loved one's recovery.

Practice Self-Care

Family members of someone with BPD may find themselves experiencing a range of emotions, including anger, frustration, guilt, and sadness. It is important to take care of your own emotional and physical needs. This includes getting enough rest, eating healthy, engaging in regular exercise, and taking time to do activities you enjoy. Practicing self-care can help you manage your emotions and be a better support system for your loved one.

Set Boundaries

It is essential to set boundaries with your loved one to prevent burnout and to protect your emotional well-being. This may include setting limits on how much time you spend with them or what behaviours you are willing to tolerate. It is important to communicate these boundaries clearly and consistently with your loved one and seek support from a therapist or support group if needed.

Practice Communication Skills

Effective communication skills are vital when dealing with someone with BPD. It is essential to remain calm, non-judgmental, and empathetic while communicating. Use "I" statements instead of "you" statements and avoid blame or criticism. Active listening skills can also be helpful, allowing your loved one to feel heard and understood.

Practice Emotional Regulation Techniques

Emotional dysregulation is a common symptom of BPD, and family members may also experience intense emotions as a result of the disorder. Practicing emotional regulation techniques can help you manage your emotions and be a positive influence on your loved one's recovery. This may include deep breathing exercises, mindfulness practices, and journaling.

Join a Support Group

Joining a support group for family members of someone with BPD can provide a safe space to share experiences and gain support from others who understand what you are going through. Support groups can also offer practical advice on coping strategies and help you feel less isolated.

Seek Professional Help

Supporting a loved one with BPD can be emotionally challenging, and family members may also benefit from seeking professional help. Therapy can offer a safe space to explore feelings and develop coping strategies. It can also help you learn how to support your loved one's recovery effectively.

In conclusion, family members of someone with BPD play an essential role in their loved one's recovery journey. Coping with the emotional toll of BPD can be challenging, but it is possible to develop coping strategies to manage the impact on your life. By educating yourself, practicing self-care, setting boundaries, practicing communication skills, practicing emotional regulation techniques, joining a support group, and seeking professional help, you can provide the support your loved one needs while taking care of your own emotional well-being.

Tips for Navigating Crisis Situations with a Loved One with BPD

Navigating crisis situations with a loved one who has borderline personality disorder (BPD) can be challenging and overwhelming. However, having a plan and understanding some tips for managing these situations can help both you and your loved one get through the crisis together. In this chapter, we will discuss some tips for navigating crisis situations with a loved one with BPD.

Educate Yourself on BPD:

It's essential to educate yourself about BPD, including the symptoms and triggers that can cause a crisis. Understanding your loved one's triggers and how they react during a crisis can help you develop a plan for dealing with these situations.

Identify Triggers:

BPD can cause intense and sudden mood swings, and it's crucial to identify the triggers that can cause these mood swings. Triggers can be anything from an argument to a change in routine or even a seemingly insignificant comment. Knowing your loved one's triggers can help you avoid them or minimize their impact.

Stay Calm:

During a crisis, it's easy to become overwhelmed and emotional. However, it's essential to stay calm and keep your emotions in check. Your loved one's emotions are already running high, and they need you to remain calm and level-headed.

Validate Your Loved One's Feelings:

During a crisis, it's essential to validate your loved one's feelings. Let them know that you understand how they feel and that you are there to support them. Validating their feelings can help them feel heard and understood.

Avoid Arguing:

Arguing with someone who has BPD during a crisis can escalate the situation and make it worse. Instead of arguing, try to remain calm and listen to your loved one. Acknowledge their feelings, and try to find a solution together.

Don't Take It Personally:

During a crisis, it's not uncommon for someone with BPD to lash out or say hurtful things. It's important to remember that these outbursts are not personal attacks on you, and they are a symptom of their illness.

Get Professional Help:

If the situation is getting out of control or if your loved one is at risk of harming themselves, it's essential to seek professional help. A mental health professional can provide support and guidance on how to manage the crisis and ensure your loved one's safety.

Encourage Your Loved One to Seek Help:

Encouraging your loved one to seek help and treatment for their BPD can make a significant difference in their recovery. It's essential to provide support and understanding and let them know that seeking help is a positive step towards managing their illness.

Practice Self-Care:

Caring for a loved one with BPD can be emotionally draining, and it's crucial to practice self-care. Take breaks, seek support from friends and family, and take care of your mental and physical health.

In conclusion, navigating crisis situations with a loved one who has BPD can be challenging, but having a plan and understanding some tips for managing these situations can make a significant difference. Remember to stay calm, validate your loved one's feelings, and seek professional help if necessary. Encourage your loved one to seek help and treatment, and practice self-care to ensure that you can continue to support them effectively.

Ingram Content Group UK Ltd.
Milton Keynes UK
UKHW010723070623
423023UK00001B/114